KICK CANCER'S ACID

A Five-Day Whole Life Detox

BY CHRISTINA BLANCHARD-HORAN, PHD
WITH CONTRIBUTIONS BY TERRY "RICCI" SAMUELS

Editing by Duncan Ayers, PhD

Illustrations and photographs are property of blanchardhoran.com

Paperback ISBN 979-8-88940-596-5

KICK CANCER'S ACID: a Five-Day Detox book about Whole Life Living and Naturally Restoring balance to hormones & liver. Detox that is good before during after chemotherapy treatment, leveling cholesterol & blood pressure also offered.

A Five-Day Whole Life Detox
to

KICK CANCER'S ACID

Five days dedicated to detoxifying your environment and your whole body

BY CHRISTINA BLANCHARD-HORAN, PHD

"The art of healing comes from nature, not from the physician. Therefore, the physician must start from nature, with an open mind."

– Paracelsus

CONTENTS

YOUR WELLNESS

Cancer Recovery with Natural Wellness: Embracing Change and Hope for the Future

Are you currently navigating a complicated cancer diagnosis and treatment path to recovery, and you are fatigued after chemo (1), taking you almost to your knees? If that sounds familiar, then this book is for you.

Hey, if you are interested in finding ways to naturally enhance your wellbeing even during chemo, renew your energy levels, and regain a sense of control, this book is here to guide you through this transformative journey.

I'm Dr. Christina Blanchard-Horan, a Wellness Advisor and Transformation Coach. As a dedicated transformation coach specializing in health improvement and cancer recovery, I understand firsthand the challenges you're facing. Having triumphed over my own cancer diagnosis, I've channeled that experience into becoming a change coach—someone who assists in health transitions and transformations.

This book is a way for us to embark on a holistic voyage of healing together, focusing on diet, detoxification, regeneration, and rejuvenation.

This is about more than physical healing; it's about reclaiming your power, finding energy and renew hope. Using a natural, organic, and scientifically supported approach, we journey together to find the answers and potential solutions that complement conventional physician's treatment naturally.

Remember, you're not alone on this path. With a little guidance and support, you can find a stronger sense of self-control and empowerment to embrace the change that your body, mind, and spirit need. Let's journey toward improved health, self-discovery, and a future filled with possibilities. Let's begin this Five-Day Detox & Restoration Program to rid the body of unnecessary acid and improve its immune system, so it can do what it does best.... beat disease! 💪🌿✨

If it's out of your hands, it deserves
freedom from your mind too.
– Ivan Nuru

INSPIRING

A Journey of Friendship & Healing

Welcome to our Cancer Detox Guide, where Dr. Christina Blanchard-Horan and Mrs. Ricci Samuels come together to share experiences with a comprehensive program. A program that came out of a unique and heartfelt story of friendship, healing, and a shared commitment to natural solutions.

In the heart of the 1970s, these two remarkable individuals, Christina and Ricci, were not just schoolmates, but were close friends. Their lives became intertwined as they navigated the paths of young adulthood, sharing in the experiences that life had in store. They laughed together, cried together, and celebrated the milestones of their journey.

One of the most profound experiences they shared was their love of natural solutions to healing. So, during the miracle of the birth of their children, their friendship grew. Their friendship was sparked by their mutual interest in natural childbirth, at a time when doctors delivered babies, and nurse midwives were rare. As new mothers, they supported each other through the joys and challenges of bringing life into the world. Over the years, they would be there for each other. Ricci was there to coach Christina before - and even during - the Cesarean birth of her daughter, and in turn, Christina (as a trained photographer) was there to delicately document special moments during Ricci's birthing experience with her husband. These moments forged an unbreakable bond, a testament to the depth of their friendship.

As time passed, life took them on separate journeys, each pursuing their passions. Dr. Christina Blanchard-Horan moved to Washington DC and embarked on a journey to become a dedicated healthcare professional and researcher. Specializing in holistic healing that is backed by science, she had a passion for natural solutions. Ricci cultivated her own passion for natural remedies and wellness on the home front in Memphis, Tennessee. They both developed a thirst for knowledge about the world of health, nutrition, and the powerful potential of nature's remedies.

Their paths converged again, not by chance, but by a shared experience. Both Christina and Ricci faced a formidable foe: cancer. These incredible women became warriors with determination and courage. Their personal battles with cancer were transformative, and even though they began this battle separately, fate would bring them back together.

Ricci's Story

Two years before these two women renewed their strong friendship, Ricci had been diagnosed with triple negative breast cancer (TNBC), one of the most aggressive forms of cancer. Here's her story before, during and after the detox.

Harmonizing Detox with Conventional Treatment

In this pivotal chapter, we delve into Ricci's extraordinary journey, a poignant narrative within the broader context of our exploration of the "Kick Cancer's Acid" 5-Day Detox. As we navigate the peaks and valleys of her battle against TNBC, Ricci's story becomes a testament to the synergies between conventional medical treatments, lifestyle changes, and natural approaches.

Ricci's diagnosis in September 2021 marked the genesis of her confrontation with a 2-centimeter mass, characterized as Grade two triple-negative breast cancer. The subsequent treatments, including Taxotere® and Cytoxan® chemotherapy, presented formidable challenges. While the initial response was partial, the quest for a complete response persisted.

March 2022 witnessed a partial mastectomy, revealing the complexity of Ricci's battle, as abnormal axillary lymph nodes came to light. A cell in one of these nodes led to more treatments, notably the formidable 'Red Devil' – Adriamycin. Ricci's vivid description of its toxicity, and the meticulous care required during its application paints a vivid picture of the challenges faced.

Thirty days of radiation, though extensive, left Ricci with a "little tan" instead of the anticipated severe skin reactions, and a chronic cough from pneumonitis due to radiation affecting the left lung. They said she had no sign of cancer. But then, a recurrence of cancer was revealed during the six-month checkup. This happens approximately 30% of the time with Breast Cancer (2). Doctors would take a more aggressive approach in August 2023, introducing gemcitabine, carboplatin, and Keytruda®. It is during this aggressive treatment that Ricci's partnership with Christina would be renewed.

It was a time when Christina lived in DC and Ricci lived in Memphis, Tennessee. They were far away, mostly Facebook friends. Until one day, Christina read a posting about a high school reunion, and they began to talk about each other's cancer battle. Christina learned about Ricci's journey, and was determined to share her research and solutions she had used after her leukemia diagnosis.

Detox, for Ricci, became a complementary force, working alongside medical treatments to fortify the body's response so that ultimately, she would have what the doctor's called an unexpectedly "marvelous response" to treatment. Ricci knew then that the delicate dance of reducing stress, a change in her diet, combined with the chemotherapy, was a potent strategy - one that she wanted to share - treatment strategies that her friend Christina had brought to bear on her health.

Now let's continue this incredible journey of friendship, healing, and empowerment. Let their story empower you as you work towards a healthier, cancer-free future.

Looking at this study, the difference in survival rates were less than 10% between those who got chemo and those who did not.

TRANSFORMING

Wellness & Transformation

My name is Dr. Christina Blanchard-Horan. I designed this program based upon years of research experience and working with people who have had a cancer diagnosis. The results speak for themselves.

I started my journey the time I recognized that my friends, family, and even I, had been diagnosed with one form of cancer or another. Then, my best friend from high school sent a message about our 40-year reunion. My friend Ricci revealed that she too had been battling cancer for three years.

As someone who has been involved in healthcare research for over 20 years, I was determined to find answers. How did we get it, and how could we solve the problem? When I discovered the answer to the first question, "why?", I realized the cause was bigger than just one person or one cancer, for that matter. I began to blog my research findings. It seemed ironic, the very industry that brought us the best healthcare in the world (pharmaceutical industry), was funded by the same industry that had dumped these toxins into our food, water and air. The toxins that made us sick in the first place. It seemed like an unintended scheme - one I won't dive into.

However, this did mean that pharmaceutical drugs were not the answer, at least for me. But my friends and family were determined to use chemotherapy. Though chemo may help fight aggressive cancers, this detox is focused on natural solutions that are helpful, with or without chemotherapy. Detox is intended to remove chemicals and toxins, like the formaldehyde they put in toilet paper, and the heavy metals the Food and Drug Administration (FDA) allows in our food, and the fluoride added to our water that is dumbing down our children (3). However, we want to make sure that this detox supports the efforts of those who choose chemotherapy, by supporting healthy cell development before, during and after therapy!

We understand that nobody wants to gamble with their lives, and radiation, chemo and surgery works, sometimes. But so do natural solutions, if given the right tools for our body to heal. The focus of the 5-day detox is to help your system work better so it can process the drugs more efficiently and effectively, and support your liver as it eliminates these toxins from the body. Because we know, based on a study posted in the NIH database (4), that chemo is only part of the story , this program is designed to improve outcomes with or without chemotherapy.

Chemotherapy or Not

One study with a large cohort that included 905 chemotherapy-exposed vs 3390 chemotherapy-naïve patients show an overall survival rate at 18 and 30 months were 76.3 vs 69.3% and 61.6 vs 54.3%, favoring chemotherapy-exposed patients (5). It appears from the study description that there was no other therapy (natural or otherwise) that was used, not that we are aware of anyway. What I mean is that we don't know if the 3390 chemo-naïve people had applied any other treatment, such as detoxing. I find it interesting that the difference in chemo versus no-chemo is less than 10%. That means that between those who chose chemo and those who did not, there was only a 10% chance of improvement if you chose chemo. What does this say? For me, this brings into question the efficacy of chemo alone, without lifestyle, dietary or environmental changes. It also means that, maybe, kicking cancer requires more than just chemotherapy.

What I have done is to combine the treatment efforts of participants, whatever they might be (chemo, radiation etc.), with knowledge gained from research on natural solutions, based upon cancer type and the available research. Sometimes, we learn about solutions along our journey because each body is different, just like each cancer type is different. It is our goal to help you live the healthiest, longest life you can imagine. Let us review some steps you can take to achieve this goal, starting with the 5-day detox.

I felt great all during the detox process and afterwards. Chemo was not shrinking the tumor before (this program), but now - with the detox - I think it helped the chemo shrink the malignancy, because it wasn't working before, and it went down 50% already!"

- Ricci S., 3-Year TNBC Cancer Warrior

DETOX & RESTORE

1 Day to Identify Toxins

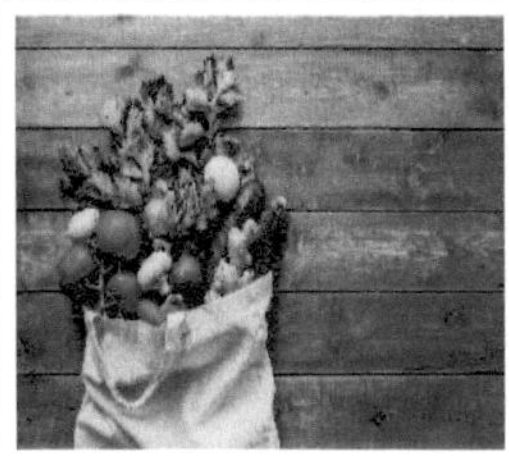	The first day is a day of preparation, removing toxins from your environment, bedroom, bathroom and kitchen! Go shopping for all of the supplies and replacement products that you will need. See the list and suggestions inside.

2 Days of Detox

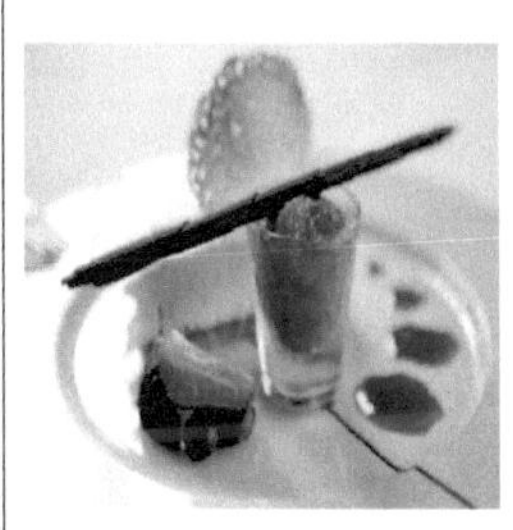	Day 2 & 3 Juice and Protein Drink fast for clearing out toxins from the body, replacing with antioxidants against cancer, and high alkaline foods that are ideal for killing cancer cells. A Sodium Bicarbonate wrap or soak will also help infuse and detox the body through sweat.

2 days to Restore & Rejuvenate

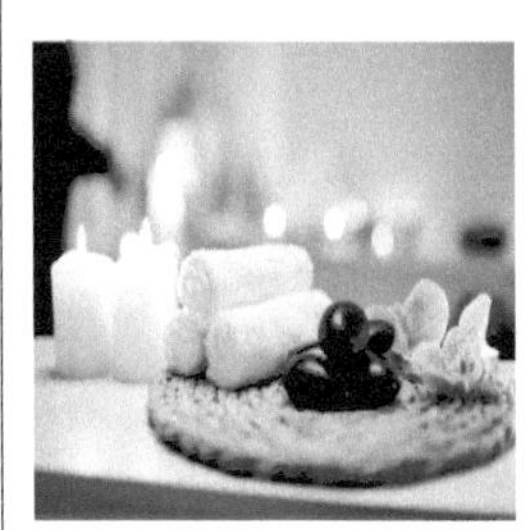	While you are restoring enzymes, amino acids, vitamins, minerals, and oxygen, we will help bring back equilibrium by showing you how to balance your hormones. Soak in magnesium Epson salt, aromatherapy massage and natural hormone treatments.

Detox Shopping List

Item	Purpose and Benefits	Cost	Notes
Beans / Legumes	Highest quality proteins are in legumes.		
Sodium Bicarbonate	Detox wrap. Alkaline supplement. Supports kidneys.		Organic Sodium Bicarbonate.
Towels and Blanket	For comfort and warmth around the house.		Basket with 5-6 towels and thin blanket.
Green Protein Powder	Alkaline and phosphorus for cell rebuilding.	$30-$40	30 day supply – used 2-3 times daily
Veggies	Dark green veggies, avocado, cabbage, and 3 large lemons more.		Include cabbage family, broccoli, etc.
Almond or Oat Milk	Unsweetened for exercises.	$4	Original or with a touch of honey.
Bee Pollen	Rich in vitamins minerals, & amino acids	$15	Teaspoon a day.
Monk Fruit Sweetener	Non-glucose sweetener.	$14	Very sweet, add after heating food
Vitamin B Drops	Cell replenishment.		If available.
Essential Oils	Lavender for nausea and headaches. Frankincense & Myrrh for health.	$50	Diffused daily.
Sour Sop Leaves	Anticancer and antimicrobial properties.	$15	2-3 leaves in tea daily or 90 days.
Wild Yam Cream	Stimulates progesterone production, various benefits.	$45 each	Two jars. Used twice daily.
Chia and Pumpkin Seeds	High-value protein sources.	$17	Eat daily.

TOXIFYING
Clean Environment

What environmental toxins are you exposed to every day? On a daily basis, there are several ways in which we unknowingly expose ourselves to toxins. First, consider this - our skin is the most absorbent organ in our bodies. This means that those things we touch can affect our growth, our health, and potentially, our overall well-being.

To remain toxin free, one must clean their environment of toxins and poisons. We should be concerned with any kind of pollution that can be absorbed through the skin, inhaled, or tasted. Basically, anything that represents a threat to your well-being.

Included in our list are common household items containing toxins, together with other things frequently contaminated by plastic material. Items like sandwich bags, dish soap, and clothes (washing soap and dryer sheets) are laced with toxins allowable by FDA, but proven harmful nonetheless. Personal hygiene items such as deodorants and lotions are among the culprits. Even the clothes we wear can be toxic to sensitive skin (6-9).

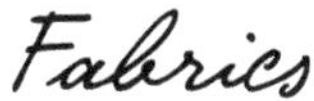

What is the science behind fabrics and endocrine blocking microfibers? I found several scientific articles on the topic (6,9).

Most importantly for this program is to remove all potentially toxic fabrics that will touch your skin this week. This includes the sheets where you sleep, your bath towels, and the clothes you'll wear this week. The best way to naturally remove chemicals from fabric is to put about a ½ cup of vinegar in a large wash load.

The best fabrics to use are rayon, cotton, wool, linen and silk, all natural fibers. All poly-fibers have plastics in them.

List of Natural Fabrics		
Here is a short list of fabrics that are made from natural sources.		
Cotton (organic)	Abaca	Sisal
Hemp	Cashmere	Alpaca
Jute	Coir	Camel
Linen	Flax	Cupro
Silk	Angora	Leather
Ramie	Bamboo	Lyocell
Wool	Bamboo fiber	Mohair
		Pineapple

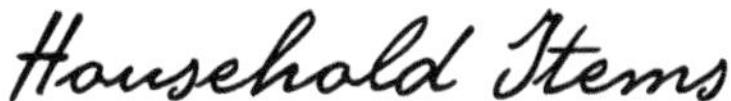

Household Items

You're probably asking yourself; how could there be toxins in my home? Doesn't the Environmental Protection Agency (EPA) and the FDA look out for our safety? The truth is that the FDA is underfunded, and is slow in moving to make change. Furthermore, changes are dictated by policy, and policies are determined by politicians, who unfortunately are known to be less than genuinely concerned about the public's welfare.

Both of these agencies have been underfunded by at least one presidential administration, who will remain unnamed. This means there are fewer agents to examine our food supply, and the manufacturers. Unfortunately, politicians and lobbyists have managed to get restrictions put in place on whether reviewers can even go into animal facilities, such as slaughterhouses. There are all kinds of rules that keep these agencies from functioning well to our advantage. Therefore, it is up to the public to determine what is safe. That's one of the reasons why I wrote this book.

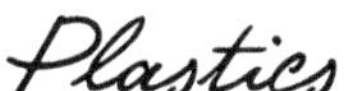

Plastics

Those old plastic bags you've been saving, especially the old ones in the back of the drawer, are breaking down now! That means there are micro plastics in the drawer. That's tiny particles that can get in your hair and under your nails.

This is one of my biggest peeves, because the EPA Knows that plastics are poisoning us, affecting our endocrine systems, which govern our hormones, and hormones tell our body what chemistry to release (10).

Do yourself and the rest of us a favor, and clear all the plastics away from foods - including food storage containers and food wrappers. Put food in glass containers whenever possible.

If the microplastics have begun breaking down, and bags are degrading, you don't want these on your skin, hands, arms etc.. It would help if you wear protective gloves to reach in the very back of the drawer (smile). Use one of those masks you saved from flu season. Breathing microplastics may weaken your immune system (11).

The department of environmental protection lists a number of items that we take for granted as safe. For example, we know that the talc in some baby powders included unsafe levels of toxins (12). Yet, due to legality of the matter, these products remained on the shelves for years after this revelation. At the end of this section see the list of toxic household and personal care items we may purchase from the local store.

Personal Care

It is hard to believe, but you should be aware that toxins are allowed in a number of personal care items. Hair and skin care products, baby care products, UV blocking creams, facial cleansers, insect repellents, perfumes, fragrances, soap, detergents, shampoos, conditioners, toothpaste - and the list goes on – can all contain harmful chemicals. I won't be addressing the reason these are still on the market, but you should be aware they are out there.

There are toxins everywhere! Time Magazine reported on the toxins in deodorant alone (7).

On the next page, you'll find a list of potentially harmful products to put on your skin. These items potentially have endocrine blockers chemicals, that is chemicals that affect our hormone distribution system (13)namely, phthalate esters, parabens, ultraviolet (UV.

Read on to understand a little better the importance of hormone distribution or skip to the list. According to a scientist at Weill Cornell (10):

"Hormones affect everything from blood sugar to blood pressure, growth Hormones affect everything from blood sugar to blood pressure, growth and fertility, sex drive, metabolism, and even sleep. Their influence goes as far as changing the way we think and act day to day."

The question remains, if there are toxic substances in the products we buy, why doesn't the FDA do anything about it?

For now, we will focus on how we can protect ourselves and our families by shopping for alternative products. Here is a list of everyday items that often have toxic contaminants that are not yet banned or restricted by the FDA. Going into the details of each of these will require another entire book dedicated to the topic.

Deodorant (parabens, triclosan, phthalates, propylene glycol and aluminum)
Hair Care (sodium lyonol sulfate)
Toothpaste (fluoride)
Soap-dish, hand, face
Makeup
Mouthwash

Face wash
Sun block
Perfumes
Lotions
Laundry detergent
Dryer Sheets
Sleepwear (flame retardants)
Cloths with un-natural fibers (polyester)
Change HVAC Filter

STRESSING
The Silent Culprit

Nowadays, we know that stress is the number one killer of humans. The role of stress in the development of disease has been well established. I found one study (14) in *Front Oncology* titled "Chronic Stress Promotes Cancer Development."

In this section, we unravel the intricate ways in which stress, that ever-present companion in our lives, becomes a silent architect of disease. Particularly, we explore how stress, when left unchecked, can lay the groundwork for the development of cancer. Let's dive into the mechanisms that connect stress to disease, peeling back the layers of its impact on our DNA, immune system, and the complex interplays within our bodies.

The DNA Damage Domino Effect

Excessive levels of stress unleash a cascade of events within our cells. One significant consequence is the promotion of carcinogenesis, the process leading to the formation of cancer. Stress hormones, when at elevated levels, induce DNA damage accumulation, setting the stage for potential mutations that can drive the development of cancerous cells (15,16)they can induce expressive DNA damage contributing to the cancer development. However, it is unknown whether stress hormones have genotoxic effects in oral keratinocytes. This study investigated the effects of stress hormones on DNA damage in a human oral keratinocyte cell line (NOK-SI.

Undermining Our Body's Defenders

Stress doesn't stop at DNA damage; it extends its influence to our immune system. Excessive stress hormones hinder the effective functioning of immune cells, preventing them from controlling the rapid growth of cancer cells. This interference manifests as increased inflammation and a suppression of our body's natural defense mechanisms, creating an environment that is conducive to the unchecked proliferation of cancer (17) .

Tumor Microenvironment: Stress a Co-Conspirator

Beyond our cells and immune system, stress infiltrates the intricate microenvironment of tumors. It acts on tumor cells, influencing the tumor's growth, invasion, and metastasis. Stress, it seems, plays a role not just in the initiation but also in the progression of cancer, fostering an environment where tumors can thrive and spread (18).

Stress, Microbiota-Gut-Brain Axis, and Disease

As our understanding of the body's complexity deepens, emerging trends reveal a potential link between chronic stress and the microbiota-gut-brain axis (19). According to a publication in the NIH database (19), "*The gut-brain axis (GBA) consists of bidirectional communication between the central and the enteric nervous system, **linking emotional and cognitive centers of the brain with peripheral intestinal functions**.*" Investigations into this correlation shed light on its impact on intestinal diseases. This uncharted territory opens new avenues of exploration, hinting at the intricate ways in which stress may influence not just cancer, but a spectrum of diseases.

De-stress

One of the main goals of this program is to find better ways to de-stress in this highly stressful world we live in. In the realm of our body's response to stress, it's like unleashing a superhero team, governed by the neuroendocrine system, consisting of the hypothalamic-pituitary-adrenal (HPA) axis and the sympathetic nervous system (SNS). All of these actually start in the brain.

Prolonged stress, however, takes a toll on the efficiency of this superhero team, affecting key brain regions, such as the prefrontal cortex and the hippocampus.

Enter aromatherapy, the unsung hero in stress management. Aromatherapy collaborates with the endocrine system, the top-tier commander of our internal superhero squad. By working directly with the endocrine system, aromatherapy can have a calming effect on the overall response to stress. Think of it as a strategic maneuver, a secret weapon, that helps the superheroes in our body maintain their resilience and combat the adverse effects of chronic stress.

In essence, chronic stress weakens the superhero team within us, impairing crucial brain functions. Aromatherapy, acting as a therapeutic ally, steps in to fortify the system, alleviating anxiety and stress by working in tandem with the endocrine center. It's akin to providing our internal superheroes with a revitalizing elixir, ensuring they remain steadfast in preserving your well-being amidst the challenges of modern life. Now let's take a deeper look into essential oils (EOs) as an easy way to help in stress reduction.

Do EOs Work?

Within the fragrant realm of EOs lies that profound practice known as aromatherapy, an exploration that takes center stage in this enlightening chapter. Aromatherapy, defined as the inhalation of EOs to enhance health and well-being, unveils a world where nature's essence becomes a therapeutic elixir.

EOs, extracted from plants and brimming with a concentrated amalgamation of chemicals, present a compelling avenue for holistic wellness (20). The power of these botanical extracts extends beyond mere aroma, as their chemical compositions hold the potential to be inhaled or gently applied to the skin.

Inhaling EOs, the essence of aromatherapy, serves as a gateway to feeling better holistically. This chapter embarks on a journey through the multifaceted benefits of aromatherapy. Delving into the intersection of science and tradition, we unravel the therapeutic potential of EOs.

For example, sometimes physicians recommend cancer patients use aromatherapy to help with sleep and to relieve stress (21,22). Consider the nuanced recommendations of physicians advocating for the use of aromatherapy in cancer patients, specifically for alleviating sleep disturbances and stress. The aromatic embrace of EOs becomes a soothing companion, offering solace amidst the challenges of the cancer journey.

The profound impact of EOs in relieving anxiety and stress transcends conventional approaches. Lavender oil, a star in this aromatic ensemble, not only aids in treating insomnia, but stands shoulder to shoulder with pharmaceutical interventions like Lorazepam for generalized anxiety disorder (23)accompanied by nervousness and other symptoms (Generalised Anxiety Disorder, GAD. Blanchard-Horan & Njage, (2024) conducted a comprehensive review of studies around six essential oils demonstrating their impact on health and wellbeing.

The question arises: where can one find a comprehensive exploration of the evidence validating the success of aromatherapy? This chapter serves as your guide through the intricate tapestry of research and empirical support, offering a panoramic view of the efficacy of aromatherapy in diverse health scenarios.

As we navigate the aromatic landscape, let us delve into the science-backed revelations and age-old wisdom that converge in the realm of aromatherapy. EOs, with their aromatic allure, invite you to explore a holistic approach to well-being.

PREPARING

What to Include?

I don't have to tell you – we shoot for a soul changing experience. We hope to inspire you to a better understanding of your body's needs, and how to take action.

Preparing for Total Change

We will be discussing all the items in this list of activities in detail within this book. This list is intended as a guide for the next 5 days of cleansing, detox, and follow-up recovery. It is not exhaustive. It may be determined that you need other or different options than are listed. That is a possibility, and you will have to make your own decisions about what is best for you. If it doesn't feel right, don't do it. For example, if you have thin blood, it wouldn't be wise to recommend Milk Thistle. If you have leukemia, we may want to use Lemongrass EO for aromatherapy and listen to 100,000 Hertz musical tones (24)neurological, and biochemical. It begins by narrowing music to sound and sound to vibration. The focus is on low frequency sound (up to 250 Hz.

Detox Shopping

These are some of the important things to have at hand for the detox. They should all be labeled ***organic***.

- **Supplements**: Cytotoxic & Black Seed Oil 40 mg, Thymoquinone, Frankincense (Boswellia 500 mg)
- **Protein alkaline powdered drink**, unsweetened
- **Monk Fruit** (Glucose-free Sweetener) and Baja Gold Salt, if not available - Celtic Salt (82 minerals)
- **Bee Pollen** (loaded with amino acids, proteins & vitamins)
- **Wild Yam Cream** (hormone restoration)
- **EOs**: Frankincense, Myrrh, Lavender (anti-cancer)
- **Soursop leaves** (Antiproliferation Activity and Apoptotic Mechanism of Soursop is toxic to cervical & MCF7 breast cancer cells (25)and the incidence rate has increased annually. Traditional medicine is frequently used as a cancer treatment, and soursop or Annona muricata L (A. muricata)
- **Probiotic** for after the juice fast – (replenish gut biome)
- **Mushroom coffee** (MUD) and/or Ashwagandha and Turmeric powder drink for breakfast

Other items will be provided if you sign up for an in-person full detox coaching experience.

The detoxification process may be done more than once, in fact - that is recommended. You will likely find some elements or activities that you would like to repeat again and again. We will begin with a quick review of each day in a little more detail.

Good to Have
Juicer
Smoothie Maker
Diffuser
Bathtub
Bottles for mixing EOs
Insight Timer App

EOs

For more on EOs, check out my book: 'Wellness, Wholeness & Essential Oils'. This list of essential oils can be used during a detox.

Frankincense	Peppermint
Lavender	Oregano
Jojoba oil	Geranium
Myrrh	Rosemary

DETOXING

Detox Outline

Day 1

- **ENVIRONMENTAL CLEANSE** - On the first day, take the time to clean your environment. Identify all toxins with which your skin might come into contact, and replace items with plant-based, safe products. Today is the day to wash and shop. Clean your clothes and replace toxic hygiene items and household products. Select what you will wear for the week from natural materials (see previous section on clothing). We suggest washing with a bit of vinegar and a few drops of geranium oil.
- **EXERCISE** - The 15 minute "3, 6, 9 Method" should be used. This means getting your heart rate up for 30 seconds and doing moderate exercise for 60 to 90 seconds (walking). Do this six times.
- **EAT** – Morning: oatmeal, or have something green, a green drink if you like, with a smoothie. Mid-day fruit – keep to a minimum, as it contains fructose that converts to glucose. Vegetarian soup for dinner. Take a ½ Tsp bee pollen & 1 Tbs Bentonite Clay – morning and night (if on chemo omit bentonite clay).
- **BREATH** – Essential oils today is Lavender. Put 10 drops in a diffuser, blowing into a frequented room. Practice learning breathing (pranayama) calming techniques.

- **WRAP** the affected area in Castor oil for the night. For example, left breast had lumpectomy. Cover.
- **SLEEP** – Plan an early night ritual. On this first day, go to bed early, and as you lay in bed, tell yourself, "I will rise early tomorrow before my alarm and feel ready for my cleansing." See what happens.

Day 2

- **MEDITATE** - listen, pray for someone you forgive, and express gratitude for your life and your breath, with a review of five things you are grateful for. Most importantly, forgive yourself.
- **EXERCISE** - 3, 6, 9 method - continuing all the activities from the previous day, removing all hygiene items with toxins. Review face makeup and lotions for toxins.
- **FASTING** - Consume the protein drink (high in alkaline) two to three times during the day (morning, noon and night). Use soy or almond milk, no sugar added. Intersperse this with juice drinks in-between. You will have a maximum of six juice drinks and three protein drinks. Morning and evening protein drinks include two drops of frankincense and myrrh in the smoothie. Tsp bee pollen (morning). 1 Tbs Bentonite Clay morning and night (omit if on chemo).
- **JUICE** – Next, juice (organic) made of 80% carrot, 10% celery, and 10% apple. You can mix this combination. Three to six times during the day, and you can drink soursop or echinacea tea.
- **BREATH** – Add 7-10 drops of lavender EOs to the diffuser for aromatherapy in the morning and at the end of the day – best in the bathroom, where you spend time with the door closed.

- **WRAP** affected area in Castor oil (6-12 hours), best while sleeping.
- **CENTERING** - Crystal bowls sound healing (if available).

Day 3

- **MEDITATE** – listen to your heart, pray for someone, forgive someone, and express gratitude.
- **EXERCISE** - 3, 6, 9 – 30 the 15 minute "3, 6, 9 Method". This means getting your heart rate up for 30 seconds and do moderate exercise for 60 to 90 seconds (walking) six times, like a restorative yoga session.
- **JUICE FAST** - Consume a protein drink (high in alkaline) three times during the day (morning, noon, and night) with almond, soy or oat milk. Intersperse the juice drinks and Soursop tea (as directed below) in-between with a maximum of 3 juice drinks of juice or tea. Morning and evening protein drink, include two drops of frankincense and myrrh. Juice is organic. We recommend 80% carrot juice and another juice of choice. 1 Tsp bee pollen in the morning. Bentonite Clay – morning and night (1Tbs) if you are not on chemo.
- **EO** - Add one-to-two drops of frankincense and myrrh to the protein drink in the morning and at the end of the day in your protein drink.
- **AROMATHERAPY** – Put drops of Geranium in the diffuser today, refill with water if needed.
- **MASSAGE** – Aromatherapy massage with coconut oil and EO
- **WRAP** your affected body part in Castor oil.

- **EXERCISE** - 3, 6, 9 seconds intensive raising of your heart activities, then 60 to 90 seconds walking or low impact – alternating between these two 6- 9 times.
- **OPENING** spiritual centers with Healing Crystal Bowl Sounds (if available).

Day 4

- **MEDITATE** – listen to your heart, pray for someone, forgive someone, and express gratitude.
- **EXERCISE** - 3, 6, 9 Method (as described).
- **DRINK** - 1 Tbs Bentonite clay for absorption of tea contents, followed by Soursop tea x 6 hours (4-6 cups), adding Echinacea, Hibiscus, or green tea, depending upon your diagnosis. Take each of these with a grain of sea salt (literally). For each cup of tea, use a granule of Celtic salt for hydration. Add monk fruit sweetener as desired once the drink has cooled slightly.
- **EAT** - *First morning after the fast:* have a protein drink, add coconut cream and two drops of oregano oil, chia seeds and add probiotics, and a banana. Add a light whole grain, and a fruit - top with monk fruit sweetener - bananas or a citrus fruit (orange / lemon). *Lunch:* Rich Veggie Broth and salad – protein drink, ½ Tsp bee pollen. *Dinner:* Lentil soup and Bentonite Clay – morning and night (1Tbs) if not on chemo.
- **CLEANLINESS** - Steamy Shower with EO dropped in the back of the tub or
- **SOAK** – fill tub with hot water, Epson salt, baking soda (26), and your EO - 7 drops.
- **RESTORATIVE** – a restorative yoga practice or Qigong

- **AROMATHERAPY** – clove EO in a diffuser
- **WRAP** – wrap affected part in Castor oil for the night, or as long as possible.
- **BALANCE** - Heart Chakra balancing with Crystal bowls (if available).

Day 5

- **MEDITATE –** listen to your heart, pray for someone, forgive someone, and express gratitude.
- **EXERCISE 3, 6, 9 –** raise your heart activities, walking, then 60 to 90s impact – alternating times.
- **FOOD / DRINK**– Continue to eat high quality proteins and green leafy veggies and/or feel free to continue with the alkaline protein drinks, removing table salt and refined sugars from your diet (using mineral-rich salt / non-glucose sweeteners, and avoiding carbohydrates that convert into gluten).
- **EO** –If you choose to continue, add two drops of frankincense and myrrh to a protein drink daily.
- **WRAP** your affected area in castor oil nightly.
- **Scalp** – massage ½ cup castor oil, ½ cup coconut oil, and 6-10 drops of rosemary into your scalp to strengthen hair follicles for growth.
- **AROMATHERAPY** – Swap out EOs daily. Let them fill the air for two hours in your sleeping area at night when you sleep, and/ or bathroom if you take showers daily.

EXECUTING

Meditation

Now that I have outlined the 5-day detox plan, I thought we should go into more detail about each of the activities in which you will participate, starting with the removal of toxic thoughts and feelings. There are many ways to elevate your spirit in preparation for healing. In this program, we work with meditation, prayer and forgiveness for a holistic approach to spiritual cleansing of toxic thoughts and feelings.

I believe the power of prayer is well understood. However, I do want to speak to meditation and forgiveness as a way of clearing away old negative energies in the body and spirit. Let's begin with a brief review of meditation.

Here is an outline of the basic use of meditation, prayer, and forgiveness to elevate the soul. But what is meditation, and why do most people have such a difficult time with the practice?

Meditation is a practice that involves focusing the mind and eliminating distractions, to achieve a state of mental clarity, relaxation, and heightened awareness. It often incorporates strategies like deep breathing. In yoga, this is called pranayama. Techniques like mindfulness and guided visualization may also be incorporated to achieve a focused mind.

The goal of meditation is to cultivate a sense of inner peace, to promote self-awareness, and to enhance one's overall well-being. The various reasons people meditate include stress reduction, improved concentration, spiritual growth, and a greater sense of calm and balance in their lives.

"I Can't Meditate"

So many people tell me they "can't meditate" because they can't stay focused, or they don't have time, or they're easily distracted. In this chapter, we will present to you an easy way to meditate without worry and guilt. We consider various options to kick-start your meditation practice with ease.

As mentioned earlier, let's just say that meditation is about taking the time to be quiet and just breathe. No doubt you've done that before. After a long day at work. Maybe you were on your feet all day. You sat down and just breathed. Nobody was there to bother you, you just rested your mind, and your body because it was relaxed. In that moment you just "are".

THAT, my friend, is meditation.

The idea of quieting the mind is the part that people find scary, sometimes difficult, or even impossible from their perspective.

Well, yes, it is impossible to achieve anything if you maintain such an attitude. Let us stay positive and note that anything is possible when we believe it to be so.

Although I like meditating as soon as I wake up, some people find it easier after movement, like yoga practice, a hard workout, or a run. At that point, your body is ready to rest and relax.

"Monkey Mind"

Of course, it is hard work to quieten the mind. When I'm working out, my mind starts whirling. "Monkey mind" comes from what some monks have called this state. It is where we are most of the time in our head. It is what we are accustomed to and comfortable doing, jumping from topic to topic, and conjuring stories. We are thinkers. Thinking, problem solving, worrying, and dreaming is what we do. Constantly moving mentally.

When we quiet the mind, we give our whole body a chance to heal, to move out of that state of constant motion that resonates at a low vibration. You give your brain a rest, and the whole-body benefits. Plus, if you've been stressed, you should know meditation is good at reducing cortisol levels and even helps with blood pressure (27).

Here are some tips on how to quiet the mind. Over the 40 years of my practice, I have found that there are times my mind wants to wander. Firstly, I forgive myself for not staying the course. Once I've given myself permission to relax and let go of the thoughts I was carrying around, quieting the mind is a bit easier.

I believe the trick is to recognize that you will likely be distracted, and to learn how to redirect your mind to concentrate on one thing. You probably do it at work and don't even realize it. All it is is focus. Focus on the moment. Focus on your breathing. You can even count backwards and focus on the numbers. All of these things will help you relax.

Get Inspired

What's really wonderful about this state of mind? Well, many people fail to realize that when we are in this relaxed state, we are most often inspired. The higher mind (spirit within) can speak over the conscious and subconscious mind. It is a time when we can most easily hear the inspiration that helps us solve life's problems. I like to write down my meditative inspirations so that I can then move on and not ponder them further after meditating. That means having paper and pen beside me when I'm meditating. Once I have it on paper, these thoughts are out of the way and my mind feels a little freer to relax and let go, and meditate more.

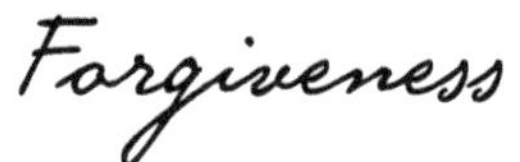

Another area that holds our spirit hostage is our feelings of anger, guilt and fear. What's one thing that can really help? The act of forgiveness is a most powerful healing tool. Studies show that letting go of anger toward another person can bring about profound change in one's spirit and their attitude (28). There is one forgiveness practice I would like to mention.

Ho'oponopono

One Hawaiian tradition stands out in this regard. Ho-oponopono is a healing process that is very simple. Let's look. Our words are powerful. Following these are the Healing steps of the Ho'oponopono practice. This act of forgiveness leads to a calmer inner peace.

Ho'oponopono Healing in 4-Steps

1. Repentance – I'M SORRY. You are the only one responsible for your thoughts. ...
2. Ask Forgiveness – PLEASE FORGIVE ME. This does not need to be as specific as step one. ...
3. Gratitude – THANK YOU. Say "Thank You" out loud with your entire being. ...
4. Love – I LOVE YOU.

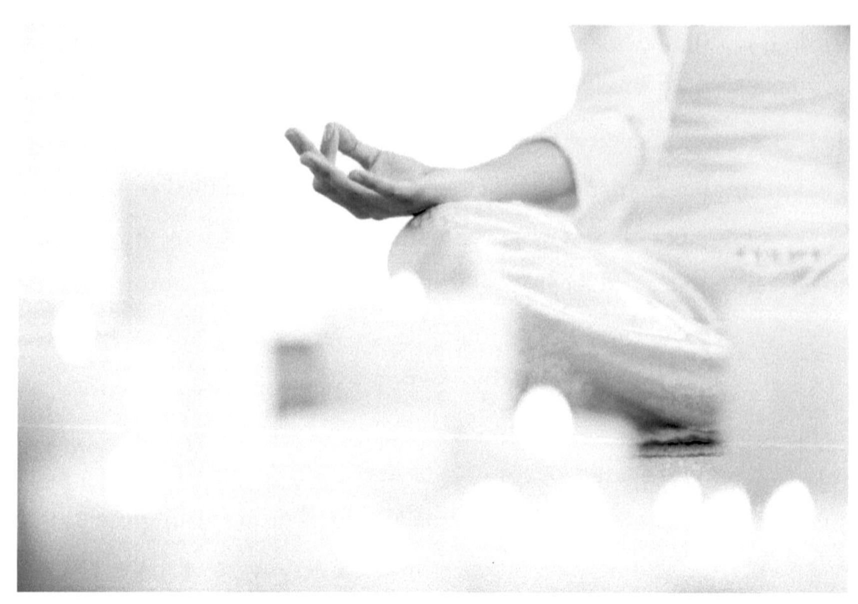

TASTING

Food is Medicine

I know you've likely heard the saying, "you are what you eat." Well, there is much truth to that saying. I say that because I know that what we eat helps to literally develop the cells that make up our body. What are some of the foods that you should be including in your diet to enhance your health and wellbeing? Here I provide a list of foods that are helpful in building immunity and strong cells. These super foods are high in protein and contain low/no polyunsaturated fats. These should be in your diet, along with some of the other foods, teas and EOs mentioned in this book.

Chia Seeds – Tbs daily
Hemp Seeds – Tbs daily
Pumpkin Seeds Tbs daily
Soursop tea
Elderberry tea
Echinacea tea

Raw Honey

One of my favorite sweeteners is **raw honey**. Raw honey has strong immunity building characteristics (29). "Raw" honey has a number of benefits. You can even put it on a wound, and it will help it heal faster. However, for the purposes of killing cancer cells, it is best to avoid honey for six weeks from the start of the detox.

Raw Honey is a gem. It is great for fighting off inflammation. However, you may choose to avoid it during fasting because it does convert to glucose. The reason I use raw honey is because it has antibacterial and antiseptic properties. Honey is great to put on wounds, cuts and scrapes. Kids love it because it soothes the pain of a scrape or cut, and tastes good with lemon for a sore throat.

Honey, even raw honey (which is very good for you) should be avoided for six weeks if you are working to reduce a malignancy or to improve a cancer prognosis.

Glucose and Cancer Cells

One thing we know about cancer cells is that they are glucose-hungry. Scientists are seeking strategies to leverage this knowledge to starve cancer cells of glucose and lactose (30,31). That is why the Ketogenic diet is emerging as an effective way to starve cancer cells. However, the Ketogenic diet involves eating animal protein.

There are some strategies that may help reduce the strength of cancer cells. The cancer cell loves an acidic environment (32–34)the extracellular pH (pHex. It is our job, therefore, to raise the alkaline levels, and to reduce the acidic environment to make it inhospitable to cancer cells. So how do we kick cancer's acid?

Avoiding Glucose-Producing Foods

Now that we know the impact of glucose on our bodies, what can we use to sweeten our food?

There are two types of sweeteners covered here. One is for the cancer detox, and that is monk fruit sweetener.

> *"Finding the right sweetener for this diet was a challenge. If you are like me, you can't stand the aftertaste of most sweeteners. I also wanted a sweetener to cook with. Then I found a red label monk fruit sweetener with no glucose. It looks and tastes like sugar and surprise, NO aftertaste!"*
>
> ***Dr. Christina Blanchard-Horan***

Bee Pollen

One important supplement is natural bee pollen, for its proteins, vitamins, and amino acids. The pollen has almost every known vitamin and amino acid needed by human beings. One tablespoon daily will give you all the vitamins and amino acids you need to supplement. What about minerals? Where do we get our minerals?

Salt

We get our minerals from the earth. Minerals are important for bone strength, for hydration, and for many other purposes. Minerals are important for building bones, muscle and nerve function, as well as regulating the body's water balance.

What minerals do we need? Calcium phosphorus, potassium, sodium chloride, magnesium, iron, zinc, iodine, chromium, copper fluoride, molybdenum, dry matter (DM), m"anganese and selenium.

Did you know that salt actually provides most of these? However, the table salt you buy for $2 is harvested with chemicals, and all minerals are taken out during processing.

Sodium is inserted back into those crystal grains.

If you were to compare a hand-harvested sea salt to the processed salt, you would be surprised at the tremendous value of the hand-harvested versions. Here are a couple of recommendations and explanations.

Baja Gold Salt is by far the best salt you can buy. It has 92 minerals, and is loaded with all three types of magnesium. So it is very good for hydration.

If that is not available, try **Celtic Salt**. It has 82 minerals, including some magnesium.

Read the label - If all else fails, buy a *naturally hand-harvested, unprocessed salt* for its abundance of minerals.

Zinc

Good for healthy skin, the immune system and wound healing, be sure to get plenty of zinc in your system. Zinc is absorbed through the skin, and can also be digested. You can get zinc through a number of sources, including food and skin care products. You can also buy zinc for making do-it-yourself lotions. Some foods high in zinc are included in the Shopping list at the end of this book.

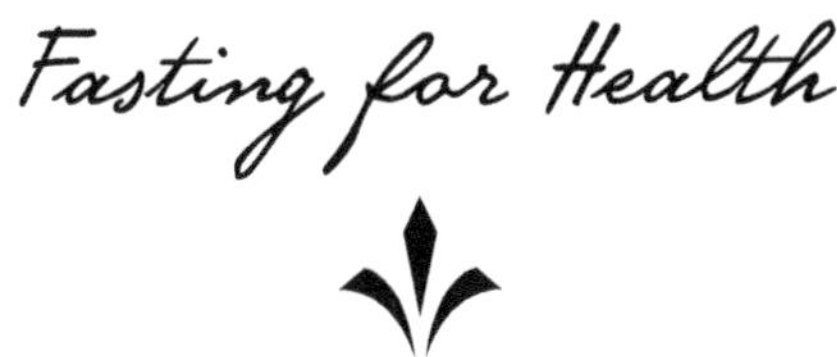

There are several different kinds of fasts that you can participate in. Not all fasts are created equal, and not all fasts will give the desired results.

Different kinds of fast

Intermittent Fasting

The Intermittent Fasting Diet was made famous by Dr. Michael Mosley and Mimi Spencer (35). I personally have seen other people use this diet and lower their cholesterol, level out their blood pressure, increase their energy and lose weight - all in the matter of a month. This is a very effective diet.

What makes this diet easy is that you don't have to do it every day. After you do the first 10 days, you shift to every other day, or three days a week.

Another Intermittent Fast

Two meals a day with 18 hours fast between, performed every 24 hours. That means a large breakfast including all necessary protein, vitamins and minerals. Suggestions can be found throughout this book on how you might achieve that.

72 Hour fast

This is a complete 3-day fast, with water or juice only. It requires careful attention as the body shifts from solids to liquids and then nothing but water for three days. Coming off of the fast requires attention to fiber and solids because the body has cleansed and requires careful reintroduction to solids, or you could find yourself with a tummy ache.

Cancer Detox

Science tells us that cancer cells love an acidic environment. Therefore, in this detox we are using a juice fast that calls for green alkaline power drinks. Our goal is to increase the alkaline and decrease the acidity in the body. These are only a sample of the types of fasting approaches that one can take to detox the system. You will have to determine - in collaboration with your wellness coach or physician - what is best for you.

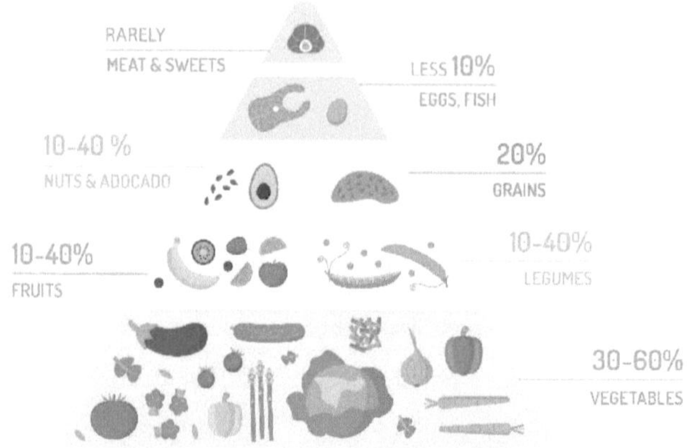

TOUCHING
Grounding or Earthing

In recent years, a growing number of people have been advocating for what is known as "grounding," or earthing. This practice involves direct physical contact with the earth's surface, usually by walking barefoot on grass or soil (36).

Grounding can be achieved in numerous ways. In essence, it involves touching the Earth or receiving the Earth's electromagnetic charge.

In this detox, we recommend that you take your shoes off and put your feet in the grass, ground, or even concrete, if no grass is available. Do this for 15-20 minutes a day. As you practice this daily for the entire fast, continue steadily for 20 days afterwards if possible. This process will help you ground your electromagnetic field. This can help your body clear away toxins more efficiently, as it will have better electromagnetic balance.

Benefits of Grounding

Have you ever noticed how your mood can take a completely different turn after walking outdoors and taking a deep breath? A walk in the woods can soothe your soul. Studies have shown that simply being outdoors can actually improve your health (37). Being close to nature - or simply touching the Earth - can be beneficial. Some studies suggest that by connecting to the Earth's natural electric charge, grounding can bring tremendous relief and stability on a physiological level (38). Stimulating blood circulation, energizing your body – even giving you better sleep – it may just be one key to unlocking greater well-being! That is another article. My point is the significance of being outdoors on our mental health.

Grounding is also called Earthing, and is a way of calming the nervous system. You may want to consider Grounding, Earthing, or just getting close to the Earth, for your health, and for relaxation.

Earthing (grounding) is a remarkable way to restore our vital connection with the Earth, and its benefits are profound. Research has revealed that Grounding can provide systemic improvements like reduced inflammation, pain relief, better sleep quality, and improved overall well-being – often quite quickly! All it takes is simple activities such as strolling barefoot outdoors or using affordable in-home grounding systems while sleeping or sitting. A growing body of evidence consisting of over 20 studies supports these effects; further demonstrating just how powerful connecting ourselves back with nature really is.

Many people find that spending time outdoors can be beneficial for both their mental and physical well-being. Taking a walk-in nature or simply sitting on the ground can provide a sense of calm and clarity. For those looking to reap the potential health benefits of grounding, it's important to remember that it is not intended as a replacement for medical treatment or advice. However, it could be used as an additional form of intervention to support physical and mental health. Getting out into nature more often can also help to reduce stress levels and improve overall well-being. So, if you're looking for ways to incorporate more relaxation into your life, why not give grounding a try? You may just find yourself feeling happier and healthier in no time!

Studies on Earthing

Studies showed that earthing can help the nervous system work better. Earthing or Grounding changes electricity in the body and brain, so it helps them to work correctly. The 2011 research findings by Sokal and Sokal report (39)stimulation, modification and regulation or therapeutic alteration of activity, electrically and chemically in the peripheral, central or autonomic nervous systems. Direct electric current or electric field alternates the function of nervous system. Coupling the human organism with the Earth directly or via a wire conductor changes the electric potential not only on the surface of the body but also inside it, changing the potential of electric environment of the human organism. Earthing refers to a direct contact with the Earth with bare feet or contact with the Earth with the use of conductive wire attached to the human body during sleeping, or daily activities. During earthing this electric potential equals to electric potential of the Earth and the value of it depends on location, time, atmospheric conditions, moisture of the surface of the Earth. The earthing which changes the density of negative charge in electric environment of the human body influences physiological processes. Our medical hypothesis states that contact with the Earth (earthing, "Empirical data showed that earthing significantly influences the electrical activity of the brain. Neuromodulatory effects of earthing may be observed in disorders associated with pain, in epilepsy where electrical hyperactivity of selected nervous cells take place, in spasticity, in movement disorders." A great argument is to use Grounding for Health strategies.

In another study, scientists reported in 2015 the effect of earthing on inflammation, the immune response to wound healing, and the prevention and treatment of chronic inflammatory and autoimmune diseases (40). So in this study, researchers show that Grounding can reduce pain and alter the numbers of circulating neutrophils and lymphocytes, and also affect various circulating chemical factors related to inflammation. If this is the case, Earthing or Grounding may have potential to affect diseases involving inflammation and autoimmune systems, such as chronic lymphocytic leukemia or other blood and bone diseases. Other possibilities are rheumatoid arthritis, systemic lupus erythematosus, inflammatory bowel disease, and multiple sclerosis.

SMELLING

Clear the Air

From the moment we inhale the breath of life, the one thing we must do to survive is breathe. In fact, I would say it is at the top of the list of the most important things in our world. In this chapter, I'd like to speak to this idea. When we are conducting a full detoxification, this includes what we eat, drink, touch and breathe. This detoxification process will involve constant exposure to aromatherapy essence oils. But first, let us look at what the studies say about the use of EOs in cancer patients around the world.

Studies about Essential Oils

A global analysis of studies found 43 investigations conducted on 3239 cancer patients in 13 countries, between 1995 to 2019 (41). The results showed that aromatherapy improved a number of physical and psychological complications (41). Due to the sheer number of areas that aromatherapy can impact, we will only explore a few of these. If you want to know more, check out my book called Wellness, Wholeness & EOs. This book provides an overview of EOs and their uses, and then focuses on six of the most effective EOs. There is a chart in the back that outlines which oil to use for which ailment.

EOs: Do They Really Work?

Aromatherapy is the practice of using EOs to promote health and well-being. EOs are extracts from plants that contain a concentrated mixture of chemicals. These chemicals can be inhaled or applied to the skin.

How aromatherapy works

Aromatherapy is a practice where people use EOs to feel better. EOs are extracts from plants. Aromatherapy is when you smell these oils. It is used to treat conditions like anxiety, stress, nausea, and many more. Cancer patients often use aromatherapy to feel better (21); pregnant women sometimes use aromatherapy to relieve nausea, and aromatherapy is sometimes used to relieve anxiety or stress. Lavender oil has been shown to be helpful in treating insomnia. So we know that certain EOs can help with various things, but where can we find a comprehensive review of the evidence for aromatherapy success?

The history of aromatherapy

Aromatherapy has been used for centuries to treat various conditions. The first recorded use of aromatherapy was in ancient Egypt. Egyptians used aromatherapy to embalm the dead and to treat illness. Aromatherapy was also used in ancient China and India. In China, aromatherapy was used to treat conditions such as colds and flu. In India, aromatherapy was used in Ayurvedic medicine to treat a variety of conditions (42).

How aromatherapy is used today

Aromatherapy is still used today to treat a variety of conditions. Aromatherapy is sometimes recommended for nausea in pregnant women. It's also used to relieve anxiety and stress. A study found that cancer patients also use aromatherapy (43)one of the most feared consequences because of its intractable nature, particularly in the terminal stage of the disease. Recent evidence-based recommendations on integrative medicine for the management of cancer pain underline the role of natural products. The present systematic review and meta-analysis aims at appraising for the first time the efficacy of aromatherapy in cancer pain in clinical studies with different design according to the most updated Preferred Reporting Items for Systematic reviews and Meta-Analyses (PRISMA. Aromatherapy is also used to treat insomnia.

Limbic System

There is very little scientific research on aromatherapy and its impact on health. There is some evidence that aromatherapy may work by affecting the limbic system (44). The limbic system is the part of the brain that controls emotions. Aromatherapy may also work by affecting the autonomic nervous system. The autonomic nervous system controls things like heart rate and blood pressure.

The benefits of aromatherapy

There is growing evidence that aromatherapy has some health benefits. Aromatherapy is sometimes recommended by doctors for nausea in pregnant women, for example, as well as to relieve anxiety and stress in mental health patients, as mentioned previously.

EOs such as bergamot are used to relieve anxiety and stress (45). Aromatherapy has been used for eons to treat insomnia. For details about which aromatherapy you want to use during a detox, you should speak with your coach, or if you prefer, you can speak with an aromatherapy specialist of your choice. The detox does make recommendations for EOs on each day.

For general purposes, because of its cleansing and antiseptic (including antifungal and anti-cancer) characteristics, this detox uses Frankincense and Myrrh. Together, this combination is very powerful. Let's talk a little more about that.

Frankincense & Myrrh

Frankincense EO is extracted from the Boswellia tree, while Myrrh EO is obtained from the Commiphora tree. Both oils are extracted through steam distillation of the resin, yielding a potent concentration of active compounds such as:

Monoterpenes (20): Known for their anti-inflammatory and antioxidant properties, these compounds help support the immune system and protect the body from oxidative stress.

Sesquiterpenes: Recognized for their ability to cross the blood-brain barrier, sesquiterpenes may enhance cognitive function and promote emotional well-being (46).

Boswellic acids: Exclusive to Frankincense, these compounds have demonstrated anti-inflammatory effects and potential cancer-fighting properties (47)China and the Arabian world independent of its use for cultural and religious rituals in Europe. During the past two decades, scientific investigations provided mounting evidence for the therapeutic potential of frankincense. We conducted a systematic review on the anti-inflammatory and anti-cancer activities of Boswellia species and their chemical ingredients (e.g. 3-O-acetyl-11-keto-β boswellic acid, α- and β-boswellic acids, 11-keto-β-boswellic acid and other boswellic acids, lupeolic acids, incensole, cembrenes, triterpenediol, tirucallic acids, and olibanumols.

Commiphoric acids: Found only in Myrrh, these acids have exhibited antimicrobial activity against various pathogens (48).

Health Benefits of Frankincense and Myrrh

Immune System Support

The combination of Frankincense and Myrrh EOs can act as a powerful tonic for the immune system (49). Their antimicrobial and anti-inflammatory properties may help defend the body against infections, viruses, and harmful bacteria.

Anti-Inflammatory Effects

Frankincense and Myrrh oils have been shown to reduce inflammation. This makes them potentially beneficial in managing a number of conditions such as arthritis, muscle pain, and skin irritations.

Skin Health

The blend of Frankincense and Myrrh oils can promote skin health due to their astringent, moisturizing, and healing properties. They may help alleviate acne, scars, and wounds, and even slow down signs of aging.

{Read more about Aromatherapy and Better Health on my website www.mystic-yogi.com}

Emotional Well-being

Both oils have a calming and grounding effect on the mind and emotions. The aromatherapy combination of Frankincense and Myrrh can alleviate stress, anxiety, and depression, while promoting relaxation and mental clarity.

Respiratory Health

Inhaling the aroma of Frankincense and Myrrh EOs may offer relief from respiratory issues such as coughs, colds, and bronchitis, thanks to their expectorant and antiseptic properties.

Safe Usage and Precautions

While Frankincense and Myrrh EOs offer numerous health benefits, it is essential to use them safely and responsibly. Always dilute the oils with a carrier oil before applying them to the skin and conduct a patch test to check for allergies. Pregnant or nursing women, and individuals with certain medical conditions should consult a healthcare professional before using these oils.

EO Safety & Side Effects

EOs are generally safe. However, there are some safety concerns. EOs are very concentrated and can be dangerous if they are not used correctly. Some EOs can cause skin irritation. If you have a skin condition, you should talk to your doctor before using EOs on your skin. EOs should not be used on open wounds or on broken skin.

What herb increases the Risk of Bleeding?

The NIH dietary supplements and bleeding report (50) stated that *Cordyceps sinensis*, Echinacea, and *Aloe vera* are loosely associated with surgical bleeding, independent of anticoagulants. In patients on anticoagulants, ginkgo biloba, chondroitin- glucosamine, melatonin, turmeric, bilberry, chamomile, fenugreek, milk thistle, and peppermint are associated with bleeding risks (50).

HEARING

Sound Healing

As with speaking the Ho'oponopono forgiveness song, the impact of the sound vibration can be powerful. We need to vibrate at a healthy frequency.

Scientists have discovered ways that sound affects our health (24) neurological, and biochemical. It begins by narrowing music to sound and sound to vibration. The focus is on low frequency sound (up to 250 Hz. Healing music, gongs, and crystal bowls can vibrate your energy centers. When it comes to how our bodies respond to vibrations, research on this subject is basically divided into three categories: hemodynamic (related to blood flow), neurological (related to the nervous system), and musculoskeletal (related to muscles and bones). For example, it explores how vibrations affect things like endothelial cells in blood vessels, activate protein kinases in the nervous system, and impact muscle reflexes and bone health.

Music and Health

Some years back it was determined that society's music should be consistent across all music, and a frequency of 440 Hz was adopted. According to some researchers, this frequency is not healthy for the human mind (51), but there are no scientific studies I could find to support this hypothesis.

So, after listening to music at different frequencies, 440 Hz versus 432 Hz. Two sessions of music listening on different days. Both sessions used the same music (movie soundtracks) there was a significant difference in mood.

The world moved away from these various frequencies when they synchronized to 440 Hz, which in and of itself is a bit odd and the most upsetting frequency. It actually shuts down the right brain according to research (52)how many frequencies are there, what are the coupling principles, what their functional meaning is, and whether body oscillations follow similar coupling principles. It is argued that physiologically, two basic coupling principles govern brain as well as body oscillations: (i.

Sound and Mitochondria

We have discovered that sound can actually help repair mitochondria. I recommend a healing frequency of 528 Hz for healing DNA (53)but the role of mitochondrial DNA (mtDNA.

When it is time to de-stress, be sure to select music that is a healing frequency. Listen to music in these frequencies before bedtime. Classical music is often recorded in one of the healing frequencies. Here are some healing frequencies you might consider – 396, 417, 528, 639, 741, 852, 963, 174, and 285 Hz.

ABSORBING
Destress and Detox

One important step in this detoxification process is a sodium bicarbonate wrap or soak. The purpose is to make your body more alkaline. This is particularly important for people who have been diagnosed with cancer, those with a compromised immune system, and other health-related conditions. Let me talk about the importance of the sodium soak in your transformation, with an emphasis on a cancer diagnosis.

> The combination for this detox is 16 oz to one gallon of boiling water and ½ cup of lemon.

One author points out that, "Lemon also has a strong antimicrobial effect in treating bacterial and fungal infections, and studies have been looking at cancer as a form of fungus," he reads a story titled "Baking Soda and lemon proven 10,000 times stronger than chemo."

Baking soda and lemon juice proven 10,000 times more powerful than chemotherapy

When combining baking soda and sodium bicarbonate, there is an increase in active components. This makes baking soda mixed with lemon juice an even stronger anticancer effect than baking soda alone.

Another study published in 2020 begs the question "Does Baking Soda Function as a Magic Bullet for Patients with Cancer? A Mini Review." In their review they explored studies on antitumor effects of sodium bicarbonate alone and with other substances (26).

In animal experiments, antitumor effects of sodium bicarbonate (in vivo) were clear (26). When considering options for particularly difficult tumors, one group of scientists stated, "The addition of some alkaline substances to neutralize acidity may be a viable approach." In other words, these scientists believe that natural products that help alkaline the body will increase the pH value of the tumor microenvironment, which will allow the malignancy to shrink.

Numerous scholars have proposed that the acidic microenvironment is a weapon for the tumor to protect itself and attack normal tissues and immune cells. Here's a little of the science. Its pro-tumorigenic effects involve local invasion (26), angiogenesis (54), and distant metastasis (55). Moreover, the initiation and development of a tumor, to a large extent, are attributed to the suppression of the immune system (56)moves toward intervention have proceeded at a faster pace than have investigations toward understanding. In melanoma in particular, many clinical trials of active immunization have been performed, and many of these have shown increases in tumor antigen-specific T cells circulating in the blood. However, clinical responses have been infrequent, arguing that mechanisms of resistance downstream from initial T cell priming may be dominant in many cases. In fact, may patients show spontaneous generation of immune effector cells and/or antibodies, implying that the priming phase has occurred already in such individuals even without vaccination. Recent attention has turned toward mechanisms of immune evasion at the effector phase of the anti-tumor immune response, predominantly within the tumor microenvironment. Huber et al[23] have fully detailed the effects of low pH on tumor immunity and the relative pathways of acidity-driven immunosuppression (57).

In essence they believe that using sodium bicarbonate (baking soda) can help decrease the chances of cancer cells spreading to other parts of the body, and also lowers the likelihood of them affecting nearby lymph nodes in experiments involving mice with breast cancer (26). In fact, they acknowledge that several doctors administer baking soda to cancer patients orally, intravenously and intra-arterially, as well as directly into the windpipe, in cases of lung cancer.

Scientists "combined immunodeficient mice with human breast cancer and administered bicarbonate-supplemented water to drink at the same time they received doxorubicin. Surprisingly, extracellular alkalization induced a 2- to 3-fold increase in the efficacy of doxorubicin (26). However, while sodium bicarbonate increased the uptake of weak-base drugs through elevating the pH, it greatly reduced the efficacy of some weak acidic chemotherapeutics (26).

SWEATING

It's a Wrap

People with a cancer diagnosis sometimes choose this five-day detoxification. For cancer, I suggest wrapping the affected area in Castor oil every night until you are healed. This could take weeks, months or a year or two, depending on the condition.

I was diagnosed with leukemia, a condition for which one cannot castor oil wrap, as it is a bone and blood cancer. However, I still do a full-body soak and castor oil rub about every 3 days.

Chemotherapy

This detox is designed to be applied before, during, and after chemotherapy. It is best to refrain from using the bentonite clay while on chemotherapy, using only two days after treatment.

Tissue Infiltration from an IV

This is called extravasation. To address the burning pain and swelling, shred a cold potato onto a sterile non-stick pad, and see the video on the website www.mystictransformationcoach.com (search for 'potato').

Skin Inflammation

An unfortunate issue with chemotherapy is damage to the surrounding (extravasation) tissue in your arm. If this occurs, shred enough potatoes to cover the wound. You will need some way to secure the pad. I recommend some simple medical tape around the edges, so that the potatoes don't fall out, and so that they stick to the skin. Using medical tape, it should be secured to the wound, yet easy to remove. This process is known to instantly take the pain down and swelling. If applied daily, after a week or two, it can also reduce the redness and swelling. Continued chemotherapy treatments can aggravate this area and may require this process to be repeated each time.

Bentonite Clay

Avoid taking Bentonite Clay a day or two before, and during the day of chemo. It is best to take it after chemotherapy, when you are ready to cleanse the chemistry out of your system.

FORMING HABITS

10 Days of Daily Activities

It takes two weeks to form a habit. This means once the official detox days have passed, it is important to keep up the good work. For the next 10 days, continue with the following exercises. This will help in the formation of a habit to carry with you for the duration.

DETOX – Don't forget to continue looking at your environment, your water, food, and air. You want to look for chemicals like sodium lauryl sulfate, as found in shampoos and sometimes toothpaste, to make them lather. Drink purified water.

RESTFUL SLEEP – Use techniques and apps or tools we discussed to help bring about a restful sleep. See the section on sound.

MEDITATE – When you rise from that restful sleep, meditate - find silence for yourself.

PRAY - Pray for someone else daily, asking for their wellbeing.

FORGIVE – Forgiveness heals the soul and allows your energy to focus on more positive outcomes. Remember Ho'oponopono.

APPRECIATE – Give thanks for what you have been given and use visualization to enhance the experience. Remember that whatever you can imagine and more can be yours when you appreciate it.

EXERCISE – 3, 6, 9 exercise strategy – yoga or another form of low impact exercise, such as Qigong.

EAT - Take in foods that are high in protein, alkaline (aka. green foods), avoid white, wheat & dairy. Focus on a plant-based diet, or at least reducing animal proteins. (See Table on next page)

AVOID – Don't poison yourself with microplastics, don't eat refined foods, especially refined sugars and salts. Foods with added salts and sugars or genetically modified organisms (GMOs).

BREATH - Alternate aromatherapy EOs every week. You can find my book 'Wellness, Wholeness and EOs' for more details about which oils are best for which condition.

Sweat – Get toxins out by sitting in a steamy hot bath for 10-15 minutes, add sodium bicarbonate to increase alkalinity.

Wrap the affected body part in castor oil every night, or whenever possible.

ABOUT THE AUTHOR

Christina Blanchard-Horan, PhD

Mastering the Art of Wellness

Dr. Christina Blanchard-Horan - her calling extended beyond academia. Driven by the desire to bring tangible transformation to people's lives, she sought wisdom from the ancient traditions of Yoga and Ayurveda. Immersing herself in the teachings of these profound systems, she became certified in both Yoga and Ayurvedic Medicine at the esteemed Yoga and Ayurvedic Center. This integration of traditional practices with modern scientific understanding paved the way for Christina to become a visionary in the realm of holistic wellness.

A testament to her wealth of knowledge and profound dedication, Christina authored the groundbreaking book "Wholeness Wellness and EOs," which serves as a comprehensive guide to unlocking the potential of EOs.

A Vision for Transformation

Driven by her vision for a healthier and harmonious world, Dr Blanchard-Horan's teachings blend scientific rigor with ancient wisdom, creating a bridge between tradition and modernity.

Christina's coaching is nothing short of life changing. Drawing upon her background as an esteemed researcher, certified Yoga practitioner with the Yoga Alliance, she is an author who equips her clients with the tools they need to navigate their unique wellness journeys.

Her approach is holistic, encompassing not only the physical aspect, but also the emotional, mental, and spiritual dimensions of well-being. Through workshops, seminars, and one-on-one guidance, Christina empowers her clients to cultivate a deep understanding of themselves and their bodies, fostering profound personal growth and lasting change.

For more on her blog post on natural remedies and other connections https://MysticTransformationCoach.com

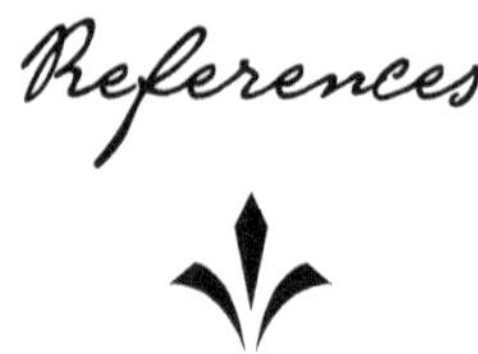

1. Mayo Clinic. Mayo Clinic. 2022 [cited 2024 Feb 12]. Cancer fatigue: Why it occurs and how to cope. Available from: https://www.mayoclinic.org/diseases-conditions/cancer/in-depth/cancer-fatigue/art-20047709

2. Blevins Primeau A. Cancer Therapy Advisor. 2018 [cited 2024 Feb 12]. Cancer Recurrence Statistics. Available from: https://www.cancertherapyadvisor.com/home/tools/fact-sheets/cancer-recurrence-statistics/

3. Veneri F, Vinceti M, Generali L, Giannone ME, Mazzoleni E, Birnbaum LS, et al. Fluoride exposure and cognitive neurodevelopment: Systematic review and dose-response meta-analysis. Environ Res. 2023 Mar 15;221:115239.

4. Guerra-Martín MD, Tejedor-Bueno MS, Correa-Casado M. Effectiveness of Complementary Therapies in Cancer Patients: A Systematic Review. Int J Environ Res Public Health. 2021 Jan 24;18(3):1017.

5. Hoeh B, Würnschimmel C, Flammia RS, Horlemann B, Sorce G, Chierigo F, et al. Effect of Chemotherapy on Overall Survival in Contemporary Metastatic Prostate Cancer Patients. Front Oncol. 2021 Nov 23;11:778858.

6. Campanale C, Massarelli C, Savino I, Locaputo V, Uricchio VF. A Detailed Review Study on Potential Effects of Microplastics and Additives of Concern on Human Health. Int J Environ Res Public Health. 2020 Feb 13;17(4):1212.

7. Heid M. TIME. 2016 [cited 2024 Feb 12]. 5 Things Wrong With Your Deodorant. Available from: https://time.com/4394051/deodorant-antiperspirant-toxic/

8. Periyasamy AP. Microfiber Emissions from Functionalized Textiles: Potential Threat for Human Health and Environmental Risks. Toxics. 2023 Apr 24;11(5):406.

9. Vassilenko E, Watkins M, Chastain S, Mertens J, Posacka AM, Patankar S, et al. Domestic laundry and microfiber pollution: Exploring fiber shedding from consumer apparel textiles. PLoS One. 2021;16(7):e0250346.

10. Weill Cornell Medicine. Hormones' Role on Our Health, and Wellness | Patient Care [Internet]. 2020 [cited 2024 Feb 12]. Available from: https://weillcornell.org/news/hormones%E2%80%99-role-on-our-health-and-wellness#:~:text=They%20play%20a%20large%20part,and%20act%20day%20to%20day.

11. Yang W, Jannatun N, Zeng Y, Liu T, Zhang G, Chen C, et al. Impacts of microplastics on immunity. Front Toxicol. 2022 Sep 27;4:956885.

12. Gondal MA, Dastageer MA, Naqvi AA, Isab AA, Maganda YW. Detection of toxic metals (lead and chromium) in talcum powder using laser induced breakdown spectroscopy. Appl Opt. 2012 Oct 20;51(30):7395–401.

13. Witorsch RJ, Thomas JA. Personal care products and endocrine disruption: A critical review of the literature. Crit Rev Toxicol. 2010 Nov;40 Suppl 3:1–30.

14. Dai S, Mo Y, Wang Y, Xiang B, Liao Q, Zhou M, et al. Chronic Stress Promotes Cancer Development. Front Oncol. 2020;10:1492.

15. Valente VB, de Melo Cardoso D, Kayahara GM, Nunes GB, Tjioe KC, Biasoli ÉR, et al. Stress hormones promote DNA damage in human oral keratinocytes. Sci Rep. 2021 Oct 5;11(1):19701.

16. Martins SG, Zilhão R, Thorsteinsdóttir S, Carlos AR. Linking Oxidative Stress and DNA Damage to Changes in the Expression of Extracellular Matrix Components. Front Genet. 2021;12:673002.

17. Webster Marketon JI, Glaser R. Stress hormones and immune function. Cell Immunol. 2008;252(1–2):16–26.

18. Tian W, Liu Y, Cao C, Zeng Y, Pan Y, Liu X, et al. Chronic Stress: Impacts on Tumor Microenvironment and Implications for Anti-Cancer Treatments. Frontiers in Cell and Developmental Biology [Internet]. 2021 [cited 2024 Feb 13];9. Available from: https://www.frontiersin.org/articles/10.3389/fcell.2021.777018

19. Carabotti M, Scirocco A, Maselli MA, Severi C. The gut-brain axis: interactions between enteric microbiota, central and enteric nervous systems. Ann Gastroenterol. 2015;28(2):203–9.

20. Zielińska-Błajet M, Feder-Kubis J. Monoterpenes and Their Derivatives-Recent Development in Biological and Medical Applications. Int J Mol Sci. 2020 Sep 25;21(19):7078.

21. NCI. Aromatherapy With Essential Oils - NCI [Internet]. 2007 [cited 2023 Dec 6]. Available from: https://www.cancer.gov/about-cancer/treatment/cam/patient/aromatherapy-pdq

22. Wakui N, Togawa C, Ichikawa K, Matsuoka R, Watanabe M, Okami A, et al. Relieving psychological stress and improving sleep quality by bergamot essential oil use before bedtime and upon awakening: A randomized crossover trial. Complement Ther Med. 2023 Oct;77:102976.

23. Woelk H, Schläfke S. A multi-center, double-blind, randomised study of the Lavender oil preparation Silexan in comparison to Lorazepam for generalized anxiety disorder. Phytomcdicinc. 2010 Feb;17(2):94–9.

24. Bartel L, Mosabbir A. Possible Mechanisms for the Effects of Sound Vibration on Human Health. Healthcare (Basel). 2021 May 18;9(5):597.

25. Hadisaputri YE, Habibah U, Abdullah FF, Halimah E, Mutakin M, Megantara S, et al. Antiproliferation Activity and Apoptotic Mechanism of Soursop (Annona muricata L.) Leaves Extract and Fractions on MCF7 Breast Cancer Cells. Breast Cancer (Dove Med Press). 2021;13:447–57.

26. Yang M, Zhong X, Yuan Y. Does Baking Soda Function as a Magic Bullet for Patients With Cancer? A Mini Review. Integr Cancer Ther. 2020;19:1534735420922579.

27. Pascoe MC, Thompson DR, Jenkins ZM, Ski CF. Mindfulness mediates the physiological markers of stress: Systematic review and meta-analysis. J Psychiatr Res. 2017 Dec;95:156–78.

28. Johns Hopkins Medicine. Forgiveness: Your Health Depends on It [Internet]. 2021 [cited 2024 Feb 13]. Available from: https://www.hopkinsmedicine.org/health/wellness-and-prevention/forgiveness-your-health-depends-on-it

29. Samarghandian S, Farkhondeh T, Samini F. Honey and Health: A Review of Recent Clinical Research. Pharmacognosy Res. 2017;9(2):121–7.

30. Zam W, Ahmed I, Yousef H. The Warburg Effect on Cancer Cells Survival: The Role of Sugar Starvation in Cancer Therapy. Curr Rev Clin Exp Pharmacol. 2021;16(1):30–8.

31. Meidenbauer JJ, Mukherjee P, Seyfried TN. The glucose ketone index calculator: a simple tool to monitor therapeutic efficacy for metabolic management of brain cancer. Nutr Metab (Lond). 2015;12:12.

32. Martínez-Zaguilán R, Seftor EA, Seftor RE, Chu YW, Gillies RJ, Hendrix MJ. Acidic pH enhances the invasive behavior of human melanoma cells. Clin Exp Metastasis. 1996 Mar;14(2):176–86.

33. Estrella V, Chen T, Lloyd M, Wojtkowiak J, Cornnell HH, Ibrahim-Hashim A, et al. Acidity generated by the tumor microenvironment drives local invasion. Cancer Res. 2013 Mar 1;73(5):1524–35.

34. Shi Q, Le X, Wang B, Abbruzzese JL, Xiong Q, He Y, et al. Regulation of vascular endothelial growth factor expression by acidosis in human cancer cells. Oncogene. 2001 Jun 21;20(28):3751–6.

35. Patterson RE, Laughlin GA, Sears DD, LaCroix AZ, Marinac C, Gallo LC, et al. INTERMITTENT FASTING AND HUMAN METABOLIC HEALTH. J Acad Nutr Diet. 2015 Aug;115(8):1203–12.

36. Ibe O, Clark S. Verywell Mind. 2023 [cited 2024 Feb 13]. Earthing–A Technique to Help Ground Your Body. Available from: https://www.verywellmind.com/what-is-earthing-5220089

37. Smith L. Why spending time outdoors can improve your health [Internet]. 2023 [cited 2024 Feb 13]. Available from: https://patient.info/news-and-features/why-spending-time-outdoors-can-improve-your-health

38. Menigoz W, Latz TT, Ely RA, Kamei C, Melvin G, Sinatra D. Integrative and lifestyle medicine strategies should include Earthing (grounding): Review of research evidence and clinical observations. Explore (NY). 2020;16(3):152–60.

39. Sokal P, Sokal K. The neuromodulative role of earthing. Med Hypotheses. 2011 Nov;77(5):824–6.

40. Oschman JL, Chevalier G, Brown R. The effects of grounding (earthing) on inflammation, the immune response, wound healing, and prevention and treatment of chronic inflammatory and autoimmune diseases. J Inflamm Res. 2015;8:83–96.

41. Farahani MA, Afsargharehbagh R, Marandi F, Moradi M, Hashemi SM, Moghadam MP, et al. Effect of aromatherapy on cancer complications: A systematic review. Complementary Therapies in Medicine. 2019 Dec 1;47:102169.

42. El-Gammal SY. Aromatherapy throughout history. Hamdard Med. 1990;33(2):41–61.

43. Corasaniti MT, Bagetta G, Morrone LA, Tonin P, Hamamura K, Hayashi T, et al. Efficacy of Essential Oils in Relieving Cancer Pain: A Systematic Review and Meta-Analysis. Int J Mol Sci. 2023 Apr 11;24(8):7085.

44. Fung TKH, Lau BWM, Ngai SPC, Tsang HWH. Therapeutic Effect and Mechanisms of Essential Oils in Mood Disorders: Interaction between the Nervous and Respiratory Systems. Int J Mol Sci. 2021 May 3;22(9):4844.

45. Saiyudthong S, Marsden CA. Acute effects of bergamot oil on anxiety-related behaviour and corticosterone level in rats. Phytother Res. 2011 Jun;25(6):858–62.

46. Arya A, Chahal R, Rao R, Rahman MdH, Kaushik D, Akhtar MF, et al. Acetylcholinesterase Inhibitory Potential of Various Sesquiterpene Analogues for Alzheimer's Disease Therapy. Biomolecules. 2021 Feb 25;11(3):350.

47. Efferth T, Oesch F. Anti-inflammatory and anti-cancer activities of frankincense: Targets, treatments and toxicities. Semin Cancer Biol. 2022 May;80:39–57.

48. Batiha GES, Wasef L, Teibo JO, Shaheen HM, Zakariya AM, Akinfe OA, et al. Commiphora myrrh: a phytochemical and pharmacological update. Naunyn Schmiedebergs Arch Pharmacol. 2023;396(3):405–20.

49. Cao B, Wei XC, Xu XR, Zhang HZ, Luo CH, Feng B, et al. Seeing the Unseen of the Combination of Two Natural Resins, Frankincense and Myrrh: Changes in Chemical Constituents and Pharmacological Activities. Molecules. 2019 Aug 24;24(17):3076.

50. Hatfield J, Saad S, Housewright C. Dietary supplements and bleeding. Proc (Bayl Univ Med Cent). 35(6):802–7.

51. Calamassi D, Pomponi GP. Music Tuned to 440 Hz Versus 432 Hz and the Health Effects: A Double-blind Cross-over Pilot Study. Explore (NY). 2019;15(4):283–90.

52. Klimesch W. The frequency architecture of brain and brain body oscillations: an analysis. Eur J Neurosci. 2018 Oct;48(7):2431–53.

53. Guo X, Xu W, Zhang W, Pan C, Thalacker-Mercer AE, Zheng H, et al. High-frequency and functional mitochondrial DNA mutations at the single-cell level. Proc Natl Acad Sci U S A. 2023 Jan 3;120(1):e2201518120.

54. Jiang X, Wang J, Deng X, Xiong F, Zhang S, Gong Z, et al. The role of microenvironment in tumor angiogenesis. Journal of Experimental & Clinical Cancer Research. 2020 Sep 30;39(1):204.

55. Boedtkjer E, Pedersen SF. The Acidic Tumor Microenvironment as a Driver of Cancer. Annu Rev Physiol. 2020 Feb 10;82:103–26.

56. Gajewski TF, Meng Y, Harlin H. Immune suppression in the tumor microenvironment. J Immunother. 2006;29(3):233–40.

57. Huber V, Camisaschi C, Berzi A, Ferro S, Lugini L, Triulzi T, et al. Cancer acidity: An ultimate frontier of tumor immune escape and a novel target of immunomodulation. Semin Cancer Biol. 2017 Apr;43:74–89.

58. Blanchard-Horan C & Njage, M (2024) *Wellness, Wholeness and Essential Oils, Six of the Most Essential Oils*. Staten Pub.

Notes

Notes

Notes

www.ingramcontent.com/pod-product-compliance
Ingram Content Group UK Ltd.
Pitfield, Milton Keynes, MK11 3LW, UK
UKHW041507070726
13610UKWH00010B/25